I0426346

The Smart & Easy Guide To Acne Treatments: How To Find The Best Natural, Organic, Herbal, DIY, And Over The Counter Skin Care Treatments & Creams To Successfully Fight Acne & Acne Scars At All Stages

Elizabeth White

Legal Stuff

COPYRIGHT

Copyright © 2013 Checkmate Marketing Group LLC. All rights reserved worldwide.

No part of this publication may be replicated, redistributed, or given away in any form without the prior written consent of the author and publisher.

Checkmate Marketing Group LLC

DISCLAIMER

THIS BOOK IS NOT DESIGNED TO, AND DOES NOT, PROVIDE MEDICAL ADVICE. ALL CONTENT ("CONTENT"), INCLUDING TEXT, GRAPHICS, IMAGES AND INFORMATION AVAILABLE IN OR THROUGH THIS BOOK ARE FOR GENERAL INFORMATIONAL PURPOSES ONLY.

THE CONTENT IS NOT INTENDED TO BE A SUBSTITUTE FOR PROFESSIONAL MEDICAL ADVICE, DIAGNOSIS OR TREATMENT. NEVER DISREGARD PROFESSIONAL MEDICAL ADVICE, OR DELAY IN SEEKING IT, BECAUSE OF SOMETHING YOU HAVE READ ON THIS BOOK. NEVER RELY ON INFORMATION ON THIS BOOK IN PLACE OF SEEKING PROFESSIONAL MEDICAL ADVICE.

THE AUTHOR, PUBLISHER AND ALL AFFILIATED PARTIES ARE NOT RESPONSIBLE OR LIABLE FOR ANY ADVICE, COURSE OF TREATMENT, DIAGNOSIS OR ANY OTHER INFORMATION, SERVICES OR PRODUCTS THAT YOU OBTAIN THROUGH THIS SITE. YOU ARE ENCOURAGED TO CONFER WITH YOUR DOCTOR WITH REGARD TO INFORMATION CONTAINED IN OR THROUGH THIS BOOK. AFTER READING THIS BOOK, YOU ARE ENCOURAGED TO REVIEW THE INFORMATION CAREFULLY WITH YOUR PROFESSIONAL HEALTHCARE PROVIDER.

LIMITATION OF LIABILITY

THE MATERIALS IN THIS BOOK ARE PROVIDED "AS IS" WITHOUT ANY EXPRESS OR IMPLIED WARRANTY OF ANY KIND INCLUDING WARRANTIES OF MERCHANTABILITY, NONINFRINGEMENT OF INTELLECTUAL PROPERTY, OR FITNESS FOR ANY PARTICULAR PURPOSE. IN NO EVENT SHALL OR ITS AGENTS OR OFFICERS BE LIABLE FOR ANY DAMAGES WHATSOEVER (INCLUDING, WITHOUT LIMITATION, DAMAGES FOR LOSS OF PROFITS, BUSINESS INTERRUPTION, LOSS OF INFORMATION, INJURY OR DEATH) ARISING OUT OF THE USE OF OR INABILITY TO USE THE MATERIALS, EVEN IF HAS BEEN ADVISED OF THE POSSIBILITY OF SUCH LOSS OR DAMAGES.

Table of Contents

Acne: What is it?

Acne is a very common skin condition affecting many people. It often appears among teenagers. Sometimes referred to as 'pimples', it usually appears on the face although it sometimes appears on other body parts including the chest, neck, shoulders and back. Acne mostly affects teens but many adults also get it. The condition is also universal-meeting it cuts across the genders and races.

The correct name for the condition is Acne Vulgaris. The main characteristic is lesions breaking out over the skin. These lesions include cysts, blackheads, and whiteheads among others, they are formed when the pores of the skin clog up.

The reason why acne appears during puberty is because at this age, the body tends to produce an excessive amount of an oily substance known as sebum. The body uses sebum to keep the skin and hair soft and lubricated. During puberty more sebum is produced than the body needs, this results in clogging of the pores, it also makes the skin feel oily.

Also during puberty the body produces a large amount of follicle cells. The dying follicle cells build up quickly and combine with the sebum to create whiteheads, this then creates an environment suitable for bacterial breeding leading to swelling and redness in the affected areas.

It is important to note that acne is a very common condition, affecting over 85 percent of people between the ages of 12 and 24. A quarter of the affected develop acne in other body parts beside the face, mostly on the neck and back. 40 percent of the sufferers deem the condition to be so severe that they seek medical attention.

Pimples usually appear on the T-Zone section of the face. This section includes the chin, the nose and the forehead, however acne can also appear on other areas of the face including the cheeks. Acne also commonly appears on the back, the neck, shoulders and chest.

By the age of 20, acne clears up in most people, however it is possible for it to persist for several years after this age. Extraordinarily, some people develop acne when they are already adults. Acne is more common in boys rather than girls.

Acne is considered to be a major problem by most people because of its effects on self image and appearance. Seeing as how most teenagers are so concerned about their self-image, acne can result in reduced self-confidence and cause feelings of depression. Some teens withdraw from social interactions while others feel frustrated and angry about the condition.

An important positive point is that acne can be treated. Those affected are advised to keep their skin clean and free from oil. The skin should be cleaned by washing with soap and water at least twice every day, especially after any activities that lead to sweating. There are many medical treatments available for acne, both over the counter and prescribed.

If the condition becomes more severe it is advised to visit a dermatologist. These doctors can prescribe various ointments to use on the skin, alongside other medications like antibiotics to deal with the bacteria that cause the condition. Dermatologists can also advise on lifestyle and dietary changes that are useful in dealing with acne.

Causes of Acne

Although acne is yet to be fully understood, the biology behind it is known. Sebum is the main cause of acne. During puberty, the body tends to produce sebum in excess. The over produced sebum combines with dead skin cells causing blocking of the hair follicles, as a result, sebum cannot escape from the skin. This creates an environment ideal for bacteria, which multiply causing the skin to become inflamed and red, this is commonly referred to as a pimple.

Testosterone the hormone can be found in both females and males and causes the skin to over produce sebum. During adolescence, the body alters its reaction to testosterone. This abnormal reaction causes the skin on the upper torso and the face to oil up. During the early 20s, however, the body normalizes the reaction to testosterone causing the acne to clear up.

Although acne is somewhat hereditary, it is not known why it affects some people but not everyone. There are other factors also known to aggravate the condition, these include menstrual cycles, certain medications, skin irritation, diet and stress. Medications causing acne include androgens, halogens, barbiturates, lithium and body building anabolic steroids. Links between acne and diet mostly have to do with skimmed milk products. Although most people are of the view that fast food and chocolate cause pimples, there is no evidence to support this.

In recent times, scientific attention has focused on the fact that narrowing hair follicles are to blame for acne. These follicles sometimes become restricted as a result of several causes, such as excessive cell shedding within follicles, water retention or abnormal cell binding causing swellings in the cells. Narrow hair follicles then prevent the expulsion of dead cells from the body, leading to their build up beneath the skin. Combined with sebum, this creates a suitable environment for the onset of acne.

There can be a temptation to squeeze or pop pimples, this will only spread the bacteria around the skin thereby aggravating the condition further. Popping pimples also causes scarring, which can be permanent.

Touching the face also worsens the acne. This habit is difficult to overcome because most people touch their faces several times on a daily basis. Acne sufferers have a compound problem in the sense that they also have bacteria and oils on their hands. Touching, therefore, exacerbates the acne symptoms. Every object that is used to touch the face should be clean, these include items such as telephone headsets and eyeglasses.

Since hair also touches the face, it is important to ensure that it is clean and free of oil. Where possible, avoid such clothing accessories as hats and headbands or use them minimally.

Myths about Acne

Scientific knowledge is clearing up most of the misconceptions that were previously associated with acne. However, some of the myths still persist. Some of the common ones include:

Myth 1- Poor Hygiene Causes Acne

This belief seems to be associated with the skin infections relating to acne. However, acne does not arise due solely to lack of cleanliness. The mixture of dead cells and sebum is located below the skin surface, making it impossible to clean. However, cleansing gently with soap and water several times daily will help to clean up the skin. When cleansing ensure you do not scrub too hard as this is known to worsen the acne.

Myth 2- Certain Foods Cause Acne

Some people believe that excessive consumption of chocolate causes pimples. However, there is no evidence to support this assertion. Studies show no relationship between acne and chocolate. This is also true for other foods associated with acne, including sugar and potato chips. However, eating these foods excessively is unhealthy. It is important to stay healthy, especially if affected by acne. This is why it is a good idea to limit the consumption of sugar and chocolate. Although French fries and chocolate have no effect on acne, some foods seem to aggravate the condition. For instance, milk, foods that are high in iodine (including seafood) seem to cause acne. People with acne should exercise moderation with these foods.

Myth 3- Sex Causes Acne

At other times, it has been claimed that celibacy and masturbation cause pimples. Again, no evidence exists to support this claim. Although there are links between the production of hormones and sexual activity, there is no relationship between sebum production and sex.

Myth 4- Acne is Natural

Today, there are lots of treatments for acne. Therefore, those suffering from the embarrassment and discomfort causes by acne can find relief from dermatologists and over-the-counter medications.

Myth 5- Acne is an Adolescent Condition

Although it is true that acne mostly affects teenagers, some adults also fall into the same loop. Acne usually clears up when one is in their early 20s. However, some people will still be affected in their 30s or 40s for the first time.

Myth 6- Acne Will Only Affect the Appearance

This skin condition has been known to cause psychological stress. Severe acne is also associated with low self image, social withdrawal and feelings of depression.

Myth 7- Popping Pimples Can Eliminate Them

Actually, popping pimples sometimes aggravates acne. It spreads the bacteria around the face. Popping also leads to scarring, which sometimes becomes permanent.

Myth 8- Sunbathing Heals Acne

Exposing the skin to the sun dries out the excess oils. Therefore, it improves acne in the short term. However, when the skin becomes accustomed to exposure to the sun, the effects die out. This exposure also damages the skin and increases the risk of cancer of the skin.

Myth 9- Make Up Causes Acne

Some makeup products clog the skin pores, which is unhealthy. Still, there are safer cosmetic products. These include those labeled 'nonacnegenic' or 'noncomedogenic'. Some brands include ingredients designed to treat acne.

Myth 10- Acne Medicine Should Be Used Excessively

Some people also believe that acne can be treated by using more medicine. However, excessive use of these acne ointments irritates the skin. Oral medicines are also dangerous if taken in large doses. The best advice would be to follow the directions given by the medication supplier.

Diet and Acne

The relationship between acne and diet is still under debate. Most people are of the view that these two are closely related. Therefore, acne sufferers are confused about whether or not to eat high fat and greasy foods and chocolate.

The Debate Is Now Over

To date, no scientific evidence exists to show that diet and acne are related. Acne does not arise from eating too many French fries and pizza or drinking soda. Acne is caused when the overly active sebaceous glands under the skin produce oil, these oils are different from the ones found in food. Although there is no relationship between the two, the myth has survived for long because most people still think it is true. Those who are of this view should, therefore, stay away from these foods.

Watch Your Diet

Although food and acne have no direct correlation, there are other nutrition and health related reasons for reducing the intake of fried, processed and high fat foods. These foods cause heart disease, which is very serious in comparison to acne.

Balanced diets with enough nutrients and vitamins reduce the risk of developing heart disease. These diets will give you enough energy and slow down the rate at which the body ages. Similarly, a healthy diet is one of the best ways to lose weight and maintain a trim, ship shape figure.

When the body takes in a balanced diet, it can perform at an optimum capacity. This later causes the body to feel better, act better and start looking better. Therefore, you need to start adding more anti-oxidant rich fiber, vegetables, fruits and complex carbohydrates to your diet. Blemish free and glowing skin may be one of the benefits that come about as a result of taking in a healthy diet.

Types of Acne

Acne ranges from mild to severe and is to be found on different parts of the body. Severe acne should be treated under the care of a health professional such as a dermatologist. However, one can treat mild acne on their own.

Acne Vulgaris

This is the most common acne type. It translates into 'common acne'. It causes blackheads, whiteheads, papules and more.

1. Blackheads

These usually occur in pores that are partially blocked. Sebum, bacteria and dead cells drain on the skin surface. The black color is as a result of the exposure of the skin pigments to the air. These can take long to clear up.

2. Whiteheads

These are found under the skin surface. They are causes when the pores of the skin are completely blocked up by bacteria, dead cells and sebum.

3. Papules

These small red lumps pop from the skin. They are tender and irritable, one should never touch or squeeze them, and doing so can cause scarring.

4. Pustules

These are also commonly referred to as zits or pimples. They appear as red circles with yellow or white centers.

5. Nodules

Nodules are larger than the other acne types. They are comprised of hard lumps beneath the skin surface. At times, they are painful and tend to last for a number of months. This acne type is vulnerable to scarring, it is therefore better to get these treated by a trained dermatologist.

6. Cysts

Cysts resemble nodules but the difference is that they are full of pus. They are likely to scar and painful if left untreated. Like nodules, you should get a dermatologist to treat them.

Acne Conglobata

This rare form of Acne Vulgaris is among the most disfiguring of them all. It causes severe psychological and physical suffering. It leads to the development of large lesions on the thighs, upper arms, buttocks, back, check and face. At times, it is accompanied by many blackheads, causing skin damage and permanent scaring. Acne Conglobata tends to persist for several years and is more common in male patients than in females.

Acne Fulminans

This refers to the development of Acne Conglobata, accompanied by joint pains and fever. The common treatment is comprised of oral steroids.

Gram-Negative Folliculitis

This bacterial infection arises as a result of treating acne using antibiotics in the long term. It causes cysts and pustules.

Pyoderma Faciale

This acne type mostly affects females aged between 20 to 40 years. It causes cysts, nodules and painful pustules and sometimes leaves scarring. Usually clearing within the year of outbreak, it is common among women who never experience acne during their teens.

Acne Rosacea

This acne form affects people beyond 30 years of age. It causes red rashes on the chin, nose, forehead and cheeks. Other skin blemishes and pimples also crop up. It is more common in females than in males, although men who develop Acne Rosacea often suffer from severe symptoms. It is different from Acne Vulgaris and requires a different treatment.

Treatment Options for Acne

Although acne is an insufferable menace, it can still be tackled. Luckily, there are many skin care products designed to deal with this. These products can be classified into 3 main categories:

- General or Preventive Acne Products

- Over the Counter Specialized Acne Products

- Prescription Skin Care Products

1. General Acne Products

These are used to prevent acne from breaking out. They include make up removers and cleansers among others. These products should be used on a daily basis as some are designed to deal specifically with acne and will act against some of the causes. For instance, they will prevent the skin pores from clogging up and will also limit the production of oil/sebum. In fact, using these products ensures that oil does not get trapped in the skin pores and therefore hamper the festering of bacteria on the skin surface.

Exfoliation products (such as skin peels) also fall into this category. They remove the dead skin cells thereby reducing the chances of bacteria developing or the pores clogging up.

2. Specialized (Over the Counter) Acne Products

These specialized skin care products can be purchased over the counter meaning you do not need a prescription to get them. They include such products as vanishing creams for extracting any extra oil around the skin. Most of them are based on salicylic acid and benzoyl peroxide which act against bacteria and acne. It is recommended that one starts with products that have lower concentrations of the benzoyl peroxide to see how the skin responds before using stronger products.

Moisturizers based on alpha-hydroxy-acids are also popular in the acne skin care department. Try one or two before zeroing-in on the specific product that works best for your skin. If they fail to work, get in contact with a dermatologist.

3. On Prescription Skin Care Products

These are prescribed by dermatologists to help deal with acne. They include ointments to apply on affected areas, oral antibiotics among other topical treatments. Dermatologists will sometimes suggest minor surgical procedures to get rid of the pustule contents. You should never squeeze or try these procedures on your own, otherwise you may have to deal with the permanent damage they are likely to cause to the skin.

Doctors also prescribe hormone-based treatments because hormonal changes also cause acne. These acne skincare products are very effective in most cases. With all these acne skincare products, it is relatively easy to tackle even the severest case of acne.

OTC Topical Medications

There are different types of OTC (over the counter) treatments for acne. Most people usually visit their local pharmacy and get various OTC medications based on advice from family, friends and television ads. However, it is better to first consult with your doctor before you use these kinds of medications. Even if acne is one of the fairly benign conditions, doctors are best placed to advise you on the best course of action to take. They will also offer appropriate suggestions particular to the kind of acne you seem to be having.

Seeing as how there are so many OTC products for acne, it is sometimes confusing to choose the best one to try out first. You should not depend on advice you get from friends. This is because what worked for them may not work on your skin. It is better to get some background knowledge relating to the active ingredients found in each medication. This way, it will be easier for you to make a more informed choice about the medication you will try.

Benzoyl peroxide is among the most popular ingredients used in acne medications. It is found in ointments and gels. It combats the bacteria that causes pimples. It also helps remove the dead skin cells which tend to accumulate on the skin surface. This way, you reduce the risk of developing whiteheads and blackheads.

Benzoyl peroxide is effective and safe for combating lesions. It should be used after the acne clears up to ensure that the skin is free from the bacteria. Additionally, this ingredient only has one side effect, the drying up of skin. To avoid this, reduce the frequency with which you apply it. The ingredient also bleaches clothing and hair, therefore you need to use it carefully.

Salicylic acid is the other popular ingredient found in acne medications. It clears up the dead skins that are known for clogging the skin pores. Products with salicylic acid should be used even after the skin clears up as a preventive measure. Using this product may dry up and irritate the skin.

Other ingredients available in acne skincare medications include sulphur and resorcinol. Resorcinol will cause the peeling of the top layer of the skin. It normally works in combination with sulphur. However, it is unclear the effect that sulphur has on acne conditions. This is despite the fact that it has been in use for over 50 years now. Often sulphur is combined with additional ingredients (besides resorcinol) such as benzoyl peroxide and salicylate acid. It is rarely used on its own because of its unpleasant and strong odor.

Benzoyl peroxide could be the most versatile of all the ingredients that are typically used in the combat of acne. It is popularly used in cleansing bars and liquids, gels, creams and lotions used directly on the skin.

Most of the skin-cleansing products are supposed to be used twice or so daily. The lotions and creams can be used as frequently as is required. For effective acne care, they should be applied directly on the pimples and around the acne. Take care that you do not get benzoyl peroxide into your nose, mouth or eyes because it causes inflammation or irritation.

Prescription Medication

Although you may be tempted to treat acne on your own, it is better to check with your dermatologist first. Doctors are better suited to give you the best advice on how to deal with acne and any other unusual skin condition you notice.

Although OTC medications are useful in treating moderate and mild acne conditions, severe cases are best left to prescription medicine and dermatological advice. Even in moderate conditions, prescription medicines are likely to work better than over the counter medications.

Prescription acne medications come in two varieties, topical and oral. Antibiotics are effective in fighting acne and can either be taken as lotions or oral medicines. Topical medications include such ingredients as retinoids and zinc.

a) Antibiotics

Tetracycline is perhaps the most common acne antibiotic. It kills the bacteria that causes acne and reduces inflammation on the skin surface. The treatment usually takes weeks or months to start working. It should be taken even after acne clears up. Common side effects associated with tetracycline include sensitivity to sunlight resulting in terrible sunburns after exposure to the sun. Other side effects include hives, dizziness and stomach upsets.

Children aged 12 years and under and pregnant women should not take tetracycline. Amongst other side effects tetracycline is known to discolor growing teeth.

b) Ointments

These antibiotic ointments tend to have fewer complications in comparison to oral ones. They kill bacteria and can be used with such topical treatments as benzoyl peroxide to ensure the bacteria cannot resist the antibiotics.

c) Retinoids

These are vitamin A derivatives and are typically used as creams or lotions. They are useful for dealing with whiteheads and blackheads se they open up clogged pores. The most common side effect is dry skin.

Severe acne can be treated using oral retinoids. They lead to the peeling of the upper skin layer, which opens the pores. These medications also lead to a reduced production of sebum.

Oral retinoids can cause adverse side effects. They may cause depression and liver damage, patients should be monitored closely to ensure that the retinoid treatment does not adversely affect them. Pregnant women should not take them because they cause birth defects. While under retinoid treatment, women need to use 2 kinds of birth control.

d) Other Medications

Acne can also be treated using certain birth control pills, in women of course. These pills change the body's hormone levels and reduce the effects of testosterone. Zinc is one of the treatments that work well in such cases. It is still wise to discuss the different options available with your dermatologist before settling on any one.

Dermatologic Care

Although mild acne is not serious, it is better to visit your dermatologist once the skin breaks out. The dermatologist will give you valuable information and advice about acne and the available treatment options. Additionally, keratosis pilaris is confused with acne at times. Therefore, visiting a dermatologist will help you determine the condition you have to ensure you do not waste time using inappropriate treatments.

Over the counter drugs are useful for dealing with mild acne conditions. However, when the case turns severe, it is better to consult with a doctor. Acne causes physical and emotional suffering. At times, it causes permanent scarring if treated improperly. If the over the counter medications are not working as expected, you need to consult with your doctor for further treatment.

Prepare for the first consultation. Write down everything you have noticed about your acne. The dermatologist is likely to ask you how long the acne has persisted, the forms it has taken (lesions, whiteheads, blackheads etc) and the treatment options you have tried out. They may also ask whether your siblings and parents had acne and whether it was severe.

Since acne treatments include oral medications, try to research to find out whether you are allergic to any of the medicines. Boys may also be required to tell how often they tend to shave while girls are likely to be asked for descriptions of their menstrual periods.

Dermatologists also offer different treatments. Therefore, knowing more about the available options will help you make a more informed decision. Antibiotics will kill the bacteria which causes acne. These come in the form of lotions and oral medicines. Both forms may also be used in severe cases.

Topical treatments include retinoic acid and benzoyl peroxide. These are typically prescribed as gels. They also case reddening or dryness of the skin, in some cases.

Physical treatments may also be recommended for dealing with severe acne cases. These include drainage of the cysts and the removal of whiteheads and blackheads.

Irrespective of the kind of treatment you choose, it is useful to follow every direction your doctor gives. Do not take less or more of the medication than was prescribed. Similarly, when the acne clears up, you should continue with the treatment unless otherwise advised. This is the best way to ensure it does not return.

Ask for information about your condition. Write down any questions you have and ask the dermatologist the next time you visit.

Common questions you may want to jot down include:

- Which is the best treatment for me?

- How fast does the treatment work and how soon will the results be manifest on my skin?

- How long does the treatment last?

- Am I likely to suffer from any side effects?

- What care should I give to my skin?

- Is it OK to use makeup?

- Which is the best way to prevent the acne scars?

Treating severe acne can be a lengthy process. Every time you visit your doctor, ensure you ask them to clear up any concerns or questions you may have with regards to your treatment or acne. Inform yourself beforehand so that you can participate as much as possible in the treatment process.

Physical Treatments

Topical ointments are the best solution for mild acne conditions. Severe cases are usually treated using ointments, oral antibiotics and such physical treatments as drainage and chemical peels.

It is a requirement that all physical treatments are conducted by a qualified dermatologist. Popping pimples ranks among the physical treatments. However, it is generally frowned upon. This is because it spreads out the acne causing bacteria and sometimes leads to scarring. When these physical treatments are conducted under controlled conditions (such as in a dermatologist's office), there are lower chances of risk. They also provide the best possible outcome.

Exfoliation

This involves the removal of the top skin layer either with abrasion or chemically. Chemical peels are typically done using glycolic acid or salicylic acid. It destroys the microscopic layer on the skin, unclogs the pores before removing the dead cells that have been building up underneath.

This can also be done using a liquid scrub or abrasive cloth. Glycolic acid treatments should be done after every fortnight or monthly for 6 months. However, salicylic treatments are mild. They are, therefore, often included in OTC medications. Additionally, they can be used daily.

Comedo Extraction

Whiteheads and blackheads (otherwise referred to as comedones) can be removed using sterile instruments at your dermatologist's office. Anesthetic creams are used in the infected areas before a pen-like instrument is used to remove the comedones. The instrument opens up the top to allow for the removal of the sebum and plugged skin cells. After that, an antibiotic cream will be applied. This procedure should never be tried at home.

Drainage

At times, severe acne leads to the formation of disfiguring and painful cysts under the skin. Smaller cysts are easy to treat using cortisone injections, these injections flatten the lesions in a couple of days. On the other hand, larger cysts have to be drained and removed surgically. Drainage relieves the pain and reduces the chances of scarring. The procedure has to be performed by a dermatologist using sterile instruments. It goes without saying that one should never try this procedure at home.

Light Therapy

This physical procedure is used to deal with the acne bacteria that are known to cause acne. Light therapy is especially useful in the treatment of areas that are hard to reach. However, it has a short-term effect mainly because it does not deal with the accumulation of dead cells or sebum production.

Laser therapy is used to treat the scars that arise due to acne. It is useful both for surface- level scarring and deep tissue scarring arising that come about due to serious acne conditions.

Researchers have been reviewing the use of laser treatment in dealing with acne. At the moment, several approaches are under study. These include burning the glands that produce sebum, burning the follicle sacs that produce hair and integrating oxygen into bacteria with a view to eliminating it.

Acne Treatment with Surgery or Laser

Those who suffer from persistent and severe acne usually consult dermatologists, who assist in discussions about the different treatment options that are currently available, including acne surgery and laser therapy.

If you are considering surgery or laser therapy, then it is important to evaluate each process fully. This should include a review of the required treatments, the potential side effects of each treatment and the associated costs. It is also important to select those processes that will get rid of the acne, not just the acne scarring.

a) Laser Acne Treatment

Here, varying wavelengths of laser will be aimed at the infected area. The wavelengths then pulsate against the surface of the skin and start destroying the large acne lesions and sebaceous glands. Laser also reduces the redness and inflammation surrounding the acne lesions. It then eliminates the layers of skin that were damaged to allow for the growth of new cells.

The laser technicians will typically vary the laser intensity to treat the area effectively. This desirable treatment has few side effects. It is also simple and only slightly uncomfortable. Additionally, no messy creams or (potentially dangerous) prescription drugs are used.

There is ongoing debate with regards to how effective laser treatments are. Studies show that it is effective when it comes to improving the appearance of the skin, even after a single treatment. Of course, there are also side effects, as with the other treatments used for acne. Some patients will have to grapple with red, burned skin that can last for a couple of weeks after treatment. The skin surface will also appear to be uneven, especially if the laser was applied inconsistently. Similarly, those with darker skin are likely to acquire skin discoloration due to the laser treatment.

b) Acne Surgery

This involves making incisions into affected area. After that, the dermatologist drains the clogged matter. Whiteheads and blackheads can be removed without surgery. The dermatologist, esthetician or nurse will use small pointed blades to open the comedone first before using a comedone extractor to work out the material.

Severe cysts can be removed and drained through excisional surgery, which is more complicated than the procedure described above. It is performed in a sterile environment using sterilized instruments. This reduces the risk that the bacterial infection will spread. As a result, the procedure can only be conducted under the charge of a trained professional.

Unless the deep acne cysts are extracted carefully, they are likely to develop into serious infections which could lead to severe acne scarring. Since acne surgery is likely to cause scarring, it is not a popular option.

Natural Treatments and Herbal Remedies for Acne

At the moment, no one knows how to prevent acne. Although lotions, soaps and ointments are the most popular treatment options for people with acne, most businesses today also offer herbal remedies and other natural acne treatments. The main problem is most people do not know whether these natural products actually work. Going through the websites owned by the manufacturers, one would assume that their products work. There are many testimonials where customers claim to be satisfied with the results. However, there is insufficient scientific data to support the claims. Furthermore, there are no governing bodies charged with validating the health related claims. As a result, it is difficult to determine whether the lack of oversight makes the products good or bad.

What is certain, is that natural and herbal remedies have been used since time immemorial by human civilizations. This is because the modern pharmacy is a recent medical development.

Through time, civilizations only ate foods that they raised on farms or they hunted, gathered or foraged. Although life back then was difficult and most people died young, they were generally healthier than we are today. The general belief is that this was due to the fact that in those days people did not fill up their bodies with harsh pesticides, processed ingredients among other dangerous chemical combinations.

So, how does one determine how effective natural treatments and herbal remedies for acne are? One can only research into the matter for available solutions. This requires looking around to find out the natural ingredients and herbs that are effective in the treatment of acne and get the skin care products that use these herbs and ingredients. You can then try these products out to determine whether they work for you.

Dermatologists will usually prescribe antibiotics to deal with the acne causing bacteria. The good thing is that a number of natural products are actually effective at combating bacteria. Popular natural acne remedies include Tea Tree oil and Echinacea.

Ask your dermatologist for more information on natural treatments and herbal remedies for acne. You can also research on your own to get gentle abrasives, facial peels and clay masks that are made using all-natural ingredients. However, ensure you only buy your products from reputable companies. You should also go through the ingredients label to learn about the natural options that exist for the treatment of acne.

Teens and Acne

If you are a parent and your teenage child has been struggling with acne, then this section will give you useful advice on how to deal with the situation. Acne is one of the most common of conditions. Chances are parents of teens also experienced it when they were younger.

As an adult, you know that acne eventually passes. However, this is not comforting enough to most teenagers, especially those who find the whole situation hard to deal with. Parents should be morally supportive and act as a source of advice and information on acne treatments. Parents should also help their teenagers learn about the various kinds of acne and available treatments. With this knowledge, your teenager will be in a better place to make appropriate decisions, such as whether to consult with a dermatologist.

Importantly as a parent just because you also had acne in your formative years does not mean you are an expert on the matter. New treatment methods and medications have come up since then. Today, most of the common acne conditions are easy to bring under control. Since there are a number of approaches available, it is useful to research on the available treatments before deciding on the best one for your child.

It is always wise to consult with your dermatologist. The spots that you have been noticing on your teenager's face and skin may be acne. However, there are other conditions, some of which bear a close resemblance with acne. By checking in with a dermatologist, you will get a definite diagnosis. The dermatologist will also provide you with various treatment options.

Also note that it is sometimes touchy to sit your teenager down to talk about acne. This is because they are likely to feel embarrassed about how they look. Rely on your knowledge of your child to reach out to them. Be understanding and supportive in the process.

You should never accuse them of following the habits such as sex, chocolate and oily foods causing acne. These myths are now known to be untrue.

It is likely that your child has been trying various things to bring the acne under control. Even though they may not be willing to discuss the issue with you, chances are this is one of the major concerns they have in the life at the moment.

Acne affects sociability and self image. In severe cases, it leads to withdrawal and depression. Ensure that your teenager knows that you are there for them and are willing to assist them deal with acne. Where possible, talk about your experience with acne so that they understand the condition better.

You can also remind your child that they are not alone, most people their age suffer from acne. Scientific studies estimate that about 85 percent of adolescents develop acne. 40 percent of teens also develop severe acne that requires the services of a dermatologist.

If you child has tried various OTC medications unsuccessfully, you can encourage them to visit a dermatologist. Medical treatments, including lotions, ointments, physical treatments and oral medicines, are available for those who seek them out. These treatments are also useful in clearing up the acne while relieving the physical discomfort that arises from the problem.

Note that acne is not forever. With time, the acne subsides. By the time your teen reaches their early 20s, most of the acne (if not all) will be gone.

Acne Scars

Those with moderate or mild acne are likely to recover without serious scarring. However, with severe acne, scarring is sometimes inevitable. But one should not give up hope. There are a number of treatments available that are designed to minimize the scarring or remove it completely.

Pimples tend to leave behind discolored patches on the skin. These are not really scars and are likely to clear up on their own within a year or so. Skin defects or marks that linger for longer than a year are described as scars. Luckily, they can now be treated.

Prevention of Scars

Through self control and active treatment, one can prevent acne scars. For instance, you should never pick your pimples. You will definitely feel the temptation to remove or squeeze the whiteheads and blackheads. However, you should not give in. Squeezing only causes the bacteria to spread. It also damages the skin leading to permanent scarring.

Consider using over the counter medications if you have mild acne. In case the acne is more severe, ask a dermatologist to treat you. The doctors are likely to prescribe oral medications and topical ointments to use on your skin. In other cases, they will physically remove the whiteheads or blackheads and lance the puss filled nodules before draining them. They will use sterilized surgical instruments, therefore one should never attempt these procedures at home.

The presence of bacteria causes pimples to form on the surface of the skin. This bacterium inflames and damages the skin. When the acne clears up, the skin will appear discolored. However, since this is a natural part of the healing process, it should be left as is. More often than not, the discoloration will disappear with time.

One can speed up the healing process using medications such as Alpha- Hydroxy, Renova and Retin-A Acids. Sunshine damages the skin and delays the healing process. Therefore, it is advisable to wear sunscreens anytime you go out into the sun.

Above everything else, you should avoid picking the scabs forming over the old acne lesions. These scabs are part and parcel of the healing process. When you pick them unnecessarily, you will expose the skin surface. This extends the time required by the scars to heal.

Treating Scars

There are various ways to treat the scars that are caused by acne. If the scars are not severe, you can apply a chemical peel on the skin. This will get rid of the skin's microscopic top layer after which the cells underneath will rejuvenate and grow back. On the other hand, in case the scars are severe, you can use dermabrasion or lasers to treat them. Lasers will eliminate damaged skin layers before the skin underneath is tightened. This then raises the depression that the scar caused. The process is sometimes mildly painful. However, dermatologists usually use anesthetics which numb the pain. After the laser treatment, you should heal within a period of 3 to about 10 days.

With dermabrasion, the scars will be removed through the scraping of the skin surface where scarring occurred. As you heal, a new skin layer will form to replace the scars. Both laser treatments and dermabrasion are likely to turn your skin red but it should go back to its normal color in a couple of months.

Acne Scar Removal

Currently, a number of acne scarring treatments can be procured. They will return the scarred area to its usual appearance. This is true even though, as with other types of scarring, most acne scars are sometimes impossible to remove permanently.

The treatment options that are available today are different in terms of approach. What is perfect for one person depends on a number of factors including, extent of scarring, scar types, evaluations of the effects of the scar on one's livelihood and one's budget. It is advisable to discuss the treatment options thoroughly with your dermatologist prior to making a conclusive decision.

What Causes Acne Scars

Like other types of scars, acne scars come about due to tissue damage. After the tissue is damaged, your body will initiate the repair process. It will also take the steps required to provide protection against infection.

The body sends collagen to the damaged areas. However, it sometimes produces too much collagen. After this happens, the unnecessary collagen will build up into fibrous masses that end up becoming firm and smooth acne scars with irregular shapes. Additionally, the acne scars will result due to the loss of tissue. This is actually one of the most common reasons why scars develop. Within the latter category, there are different scar types including atrophic macules, soft scars, depressed scars and the well known ice pick scars among others.

Available Treatment Options

One of the effective methods that work for most people involves the injection of collagen into scar sites. However, this has to be repeated at regular intervals- about after every 3 to 6 months. After the injection, the collagen will puff out the scarred area, thus making it almost impossible to notice the scar.

Another process involves injecting your body fat into the affected area through what is commonly known as autologus fat transfer. Fat is taken from one part of your body and injected into acne scars, thus filling it out. As with the first process, this option should also be repeated, albeit less frequently, this is because the fat will be absorbed back into your skin.

You may opt to use dermabrasion as your treatment option of choice. It is commonly performed under local anesthesia. For this procedure, thin layers of surface skin will be removed using a brush or fraise set at high speed. The process sometimes removes part of the shallow scarring from the skin surface. It also lessens the depth to which deeper scarring has occurred. Alternatively, you can go with Micro dermabrasion, here the surface skin will be removed using aluminum oxide crystals that are passed through a vacuum.

The other treatment for acne scars involves the use of lasers. The dermatologist will aim lasers of varying wavelength and intensity to the scarring to change the shape of the scars. Depending on your scars, it is possible to achieve permanent results. However, multiple treatments are sometimes required.

You also have the option of relying on skin surgery and skin grafting to treat acne scars. These procedures are reserved for extreme situations and deep scarring because they are a bit extreme.

Skin Care and Acne

Although skin care should be part of your everyday routine, it is especially important for those who have acne. To bring acne under control, you need to keep your skin as healthy as you possibly can. This involves cleaning your skin and protecting it against sources of damage such as harsh cosmetics and sunshine.

Cleaning the Skin

Ensure you use specialized skin cleaners and gentle soaps to wash your face several times daily. However, you should not scrub the skin otherwise you will aggravate the acne further. Use a soft cleaning cloth to moisten your face before applying the cleanser evenly, rinse the cleanser off with lots of water and dry off using a soft towel.

If your skin is especially oily, you should consider using an astringent. Do this carefully, applying it to those parts of your face that are the oiliest. If it irritates your skin, discontinue use. It is also important to ask your dermatologist for advice before you start using the astringent.

Additionally, you need to take good care of your hair. This is part and parcel of good skin care. Use shampoo on your hair 2 or 3 times weekly taking care that it does not drip to your face. If you have oily hair, shampoo it on a daily basis.

Sun Protection

Suntans will dry out the skin and conceal the acne, albeit temporarily. When your skin gets accustomed to the sun, the acne is likely to flare up. Suntans also come with the risk of skin damage which leads to premature ageing and, at times, causes cancer. Some of the acne medications make the skin more sensitive to sun rays and burning. Therefore, you should wear a sunscreen whenever you go out.

Choosing Makeup

To ensure your skin looks flawlessly perfect, you should discontinue your use of makeup. If you absolutely have to wear makeup, choose noncomedogenic. These special makeup products do not clog the skin pores. However, they may cause an outbreak of acne. You should also avoid using makeup that has an oil base. Always read the labels on the products carefully and use the least amount possible.

Shaving

For the best shave, use both safety razors and electric razors before you settle on the one you deem most comfortable. If the safety razor has dull blades, dispose of it and get a new one. Change the blade after 2 or 3 shaves. If your skin is blemished, shave around the blemishes. This way, you will not cut them. Before shaving, soften your beard with shaving cream and water. If there are lots of breakouts, don't shave until the bumps subside.

More on Skin Care

Try as much as possible not to touch the skin. You will definitely be tempted to pop and squeeze those pimples, you should never give in. The pimple causing bacteria will spread if you pop the acne bumps and may also cause permanent scarring.

You should also not touch the face. Most people do it subconsciously, but the hands are oily and dirty and will spread germs on the skin.

It is possible to bring acne under control. You can use medications to clear the skin up and combat the acne causing bacteria. You should aid the process by ensuring your skin is well taken care of.

Makeup and Acne

If you find yourself in a situation where you need to look perfect, you do not have to wait until the skin care products work their magic on your acne. In such a case, there are a number of creative makeup concealing tricks that will leave your face looking stunning. Keep in mind that makeup will conceal the acne, not cure it. Additionally, it is easy to conceal acne using makeup. To do this, follow these rules:

The basic acne hiding weapons you need include a finishing powder, a foundation and a concealer. Only use brand names you trust to perform the operation. Choose oil free and hypoallergenic products that are a match with your skin tone. Read the label and ensure you buy the right products. If you are using the brand for the first time, test it by applying a small dab to spots under your jaw and check if your skin reacts. Wait for an hour to see if the product reacts with your skin.

1. Starting Out

Use a normal face cleanser to wash and then dry it. Apply the acne medication as instructed and wait until it dries up.

2. The Concealer

In a light dabbing motion, apply the concealer sparingly to any red areas or dark blotches caused by the acne. Use a facial sponge to blend the concealer in. If you need to, use more concealer, do this carefully otherwise it will look terrible after it dries.

3. The Foundation

Next use foundation sparingly in a light, dabbing motion. Use a sponge to blend the foundation. Reapply as needed.

4. The Final Touch

Finally, apply oil free powder using a makeup brush. This eliminates any shine caused by the foundation and acne concealer. It will also give you that enviable finished look.

Toss out the disposable sponges so that you do not transfer the skin oil to your clean face later.

Before Bed

Thoroughly wash your face to get the makeup off before you get into bed, or immediately after you get home. This allows your skin space to breathe and airs out the acne.

Pregnancy, Birth Control Pills and Acne

Usually, acne will first break out during the teen years when the hormone levels start surging. This pushes the sebaceous glands into overdrive. They produce excess sebaceous oils that sometimes clog inside the glands. Acne then develops because the oils cannot escape.

Since fluctuating hormone levels trigger excessive production of sebaceous oils, it follows that whenever your body's hormone level alters, there are chances that acne will break out. For women, acne flare-ups are normal during pregnancy and while under birth control pills.

Controlling Acne using Birth Control Pills

If you are on these pills and you notice that your acne is worsening, consult your doctor. By switching to other brands, you can control the acne situation. This is why some women who experience moderate acne sometimes choose to use birth control pills to clear up the spots.

Healthy women above the age of 15 and who are already menstruating can decide to use oral contraceptives. If you fall into this bracket, you are allowed to get prescriptions for birth control pills from your doctor. Several brands exist that can help deal with acne. However, at the moment, only one is FDA approved for the treatment of acne. The said product is Ortho Tri-cyclen.

You should only use birth control pills to treat acne after you have exhausted the other acne treatment options. Some of the pills have side effects, therefore you must use them as prescribed.

Pregnancy and Acne

Some women also report an outbreak in acne when they are expecting a child. To prepare the body for the baby, the body sometimes changes in a number of ways.

The two main hormones working in the female body are estrogen and progesterone. During pregnancy, the progesterone becomes dominant and takes on other roles while the fetus is developing. However, estrogen is less androgenic than progesterone. This means that progesterone somewhat resembles the hormones found in the male body. Increased progesterone causes the excessive production of sebaceous oils, leading to acne.

Where possible, you can handle acne while pregnant by accepting the fact that this is a natural and temporary process. The acne usually clears up once your baby is delivered. If you still need to bring the situation under control, you should discuss the options with your dermatologist, especially one experienced in working with patients who contracted acne during pregnancy. Once you discuss the situation, your dermatologist will suggest appropriate treatment options that will not harm the baby.

Back Acne

Although you will not see it, you should be able to feel back acne. Although it affects a small percentage of the human population, it is so common that it has been nicknamed 'bacne'.

The back has many sebaceous glands that produce lots of oil. The biggest instigators of bacne include tight fitting clothes and clothing that is made using fabrics which do not give the skin space to breathe. Sometimes, wearing a backpack triggers bouts of acne. These accessories trap the oil that is produced constantly from the back's sebaceous glands. When the glands clog up, dead skin cells will be trapped within the hair follicles. After some time, bacteria forms and inflames the tissue surrounding the area. This causes acne.

All types of acne can spread out on your back, including blackheads and whiteheads, papules and pustules. Sometimes, you will also develop acne cysts when the acne forms deep within the skin.

Bacne is not triggered by poor diet, stress or hereditary factors. However, long hair does aggravate the pores. If you have back acne and long hair, it may be a good idea to keep it off your back or trim it.

Treating Back Acne

The skin on your back is thicker than that on the other body parts where acne is likely to appear. Due to the difference in the skin thickness, the treatment options for the back acne are a bit different.

You should still keep your back as clean as possible. Take showers on a frequent basis especially after you work out. Additionally, you should use cleansers that have glycolic or salicylic acid. If you have never used a loofah before, you should learn how to use one gently to remove the dead skin cells. This process is also referred to as exfoliating.

After you wash and dry the skin, ensure you apply topical products that contain benzoyl peroxide all over the back, especially to the areas that were affected by acne. Ensure that the product fully absorbs into the skin (sometimes it stains clothing). Additionally, you should only treat those areas that actually have acne, in comparison to slathering the topical product everywhere on your body. If you are not careful, your back will become too dry. If this happens, you will have to use a moisturizer. This may cause another acne breakout. In case you have problems reaching the affected areas, get someone to apply the product.

This is all you need to know about back acne and its treatment. If you do not wash your back properly, you should start doing so and you will notice almost immediate results. If the back acne gets out of hand, consult a doctor.

Scalp Acne

Most people know what acne is. It is also common knowledge that acne appears on the back, arms, chest and face. Acne also breaks out on other body parts. However, very few people know about this. Seeing as how acne is a skin condition, it is important to note that it can appear in just about any part of the body. One of these lesser known areas is the scalp.

The mildest form of scalp acne is Scalp Folliculitis. It is one of the most common conditions related to the scalp. This acne form is often triggered by stress. It irritates the scalp and develops when the scalp is oilier than normal, such as when one uses oily hair care products or fails to wash their hair frequently.

Scalp acne is also itchy and difficult to leave alone. Scalp Folliculitis causes small, sore and crusty pustules. These mostly appear at the hairline on the upper part of the forehead. There can be a couple or lots of pustules.

Acne necrotica miliaris is a more severe kind of scalp acne. It is characterized by large, inflamed papules with black colored crusts. This acne variety leaves scars behind similar to those caused by Chicken Pox.

Another severe variety of scalp acne mostly affects adult African-American men, but can affect just about anyone else. This rare condition involves a combination of small pustules and papules and large cysts. With time, the papules and pustules grow in size.

Treating Scalp Acne

You can treat mild scalp acne using the usual acne medications and treatment options. Use products that contain salicylic acid to clean the affected area. Since these products tend to cause excessive dryness, you should only use them on the affected areas. The best way to do this would be to use a cotton ball to apply the medication. Also, since oily hair sometimes contributes to the development of scalp acne, you should shampoo often. Use shampoos that have been formulated for your kind of hair. Most of the hair care products that are designed to treat seborrhea are also useful in treating scalp acne. If you plan on applying any other product on your hair (such as a hair gel), ensure you read the label so that you do not end up with more acne.

If the scalp acne is particularly severe, consult your dermatologist or doctor first before you attempt any treatment option. Similarly, you should never use any product that has benzoyl peroxide to treat the acne on your scalp. When peroxide touches the hair, it can change its color, resulting in undesirable effects. If you chemically textured your hair (for instance with a perm), or color treated it, you are at a higher risk of experiencing trouble with your hair if you use products with benzoyl peroxide.

Acne in Young People and Babies

Should you notice acne on your infant's body, do not panic. This is quite normal. The acne should clear up on its own and will rarely require the use of medications or dermatological consultations.

Babies, newborns especially, often develop acne bumps due to the trapping of skin oil in the hair follicles. Most of the acne breaks out on the cheeks, chin and forehead.

After noticing the acne, bathe the baby as you usually do. Use a soft and clean washcloth with ordinary hypoallergenic baby soap. If the condition worsens or fails to clear up after a couple of weeks, check with your doctor for further advice.

Acne Issues in Teens

Occasional blemishes start out on most people, irrespective of age. However, persistent acne normally breaks out when one reaches puberty. You should discard all the myths that connect oily foods and chocolate to acne. Similarly, it is not related to failing to wash your face on a regular basis. Washing the face too much will clog the pores, irritate the skin and cause a more severe acne breakout.

Prevention and Treatment of Acne in Children

Although it is not possible to prevent acne, there are measures you can take to reduce how the acne appears. Encourage your child to wash gently twice a day, using mild hypoallergenic soaps, soft facecloths and warm water.

In case your daughter already wears makeup, ask her to choose noncomedogenic cosmetics. Unlike the rest, these products cannot promote acne. Similarly, advise her to always remove her makeup the moment she gets home. Of course, you should not forget to remind her that popping the pimples will only make things worse.

Over the counter products manufactured using benzoyl peroxide are useful in treating acne. These products include crèmes and lotions from different manufacturers. You can save money through a simple comparison between national brands and store brands. In case the ingredients are similar and at the same level, choose the cheaper ones.

The percentage of benzoyl peroxide differs in the various brands. Choose products that have higher concentrations. You should also test the products on your child to check whether there are any unsavory reactions.

If the products do not cause any significant improvement within a month or 6 weeks after you started the treatment, visit a regular doctor with your child for further medical examinations. Ask the doctor for treatment advice. Unless the doctor recommends it, you should not head to a dermatologist.

Acne in children can break out at any time. Ensure you are there to provide the physical, monetary and emotional support your child needs to go through the stigma that arises from acne. The problem is usually of a bigger deal to children than it is to adults.

We Want Your Feedback on This Book!

Our main purpose is to make sure that our readers get value from the books we publish and that they have a good experience with all of our products. We are always working to improve our books and other products with every revision and update.

Every piece of feedback makes a difference in this process. And we would appreciate yours as well - whether it is good or bad.

Please take one minute to let us know what you thought by following this link:

http://checkmatemg.com/feedbackacne/

www.ingramcontent.com/pod-product-compliance
Lightning Source LLC
Chambersburg PA
CBHW070818290526
45795CB00002B/751